I0421497

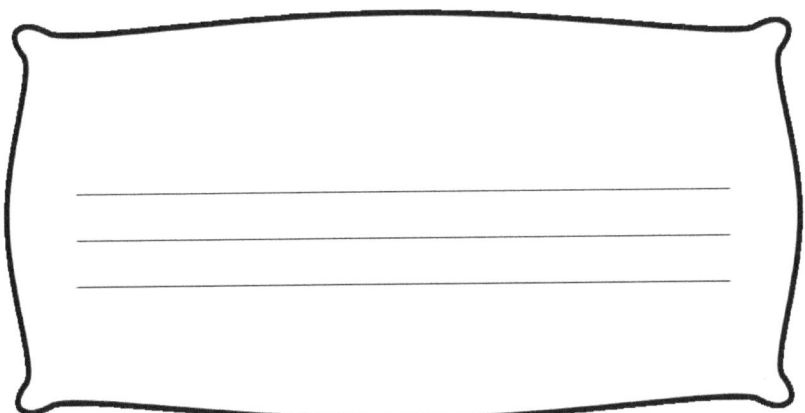

Daily Food Diary

Date

Breakfast
Time:

Calories/
Points:

Lunch
Time:

Calories/
Points:

Dinner
Time:

Calories/
Points:

Snack 1
Time:

Calories/
Points:

Snack 2
Time:

Calories/
Points:

Vitamins

Veggies & Fruits

Water

Today's Workout

Stats
Total
Calories/Points:

Fat:

Fiber:

Carbs:

Protein:

Exercise:

Sleep:

Notes

Daily Food Diary

Date _____

Breakfast	*Lunch*	*Dinner*	*Snack 1*	*Snack 2*
Time:	Time:	Time:	Time:	Time:

Calories/Points: Calories/Points: Calories/Points: Calories/Points: Calories/Points:

Vitamins

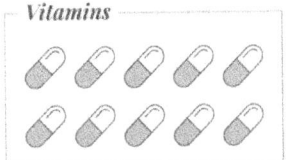

Veggies & Fruits

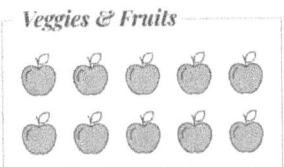

Water

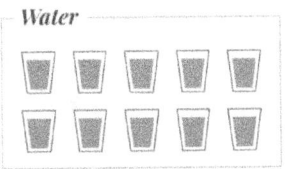

Today's Workout

Stats

Total Calories/Points:

Fat:

Fiber:

Carbs:

Protein:

Exercise:

Sleep:

Notes

Daily Food Diary

Date

Breakfast
Time:

Calories/
Points:

Lunch
Time:

Calories/
Points:

Dinner
Time:

Calories/
Points:

Snack 1
Time:

Calories/
Points:

Snack 2
Time:

Calories/
Points:

Vitamins

Veggies & Fruits

Water

Today's Workout

Stats

Total
Calories/Points:

Fat:

Fiber:

Carbs:

Protein:

Exercise:

Sleep:

Notes

Daily Food Diary

Date

Breakfast
Time:

....
....
....
....
....
....
....
....
....
....
....
....
....
....
....
....
....

Calories/
Points:

Lunch
Time:

....
....
....
....
....
....
....
....
....
....
....
....
....
....
....
....
....

Calories/
Points:

Dinner
Time:

....
....
....
....
....
....
....
....
....
....
....
....
....
....
....
....
....

Calories/
Points:

Snack 1
Time:

....
....
....
....
....
....
....
....
....
....
....
....
....
....
....
....
....

Calories/
Points:

Snack 2
Time:

....
....
....
....
....
....
....
....
....
....
....
....
....
....
....
....
....

Calories/
Points:

Vitamins
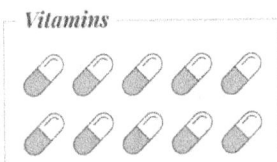

Veggies & Fruits
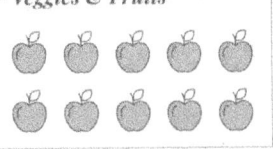

Water
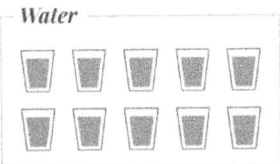

Today's Workout
....
....
....
....
....
....
....

Stats
Total
Calories/Points:

Fat:

Fiber:

Carbs:

Protein:

Exercise:

Sleep:

Notes
....
....
....
....
....
....

Daily Food Diary

Date

Breakfast
Time:

Calories/
Points:

Lunch
Time:

Calories/
Points:

Dinner
Time:

Calories/
Points:

Snack 1
Time:

Calories/
Points:

Snack 2
Time:

Calories/
Points:

Vitamins

Veggies & Fruits

Water

Today's Workout

Stats

Total
Calories/Points:

Fat:

Fiber:

Carbs:

Protein:

Exercise:

Sleep:

Notes

Daily Food Diary

Date

Breakfast	Lunch	Dinner	Snack 1	Snack 2
Time:	Time:	Time:	Time:	Time:
Calories/ Points:	Calories/ Points:	Calories/ Points:	Calories/ Points:	Calories/ Points:

Vitamins

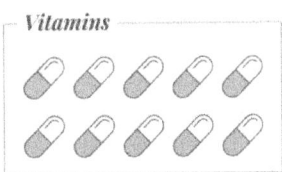

Veggies & Fruits

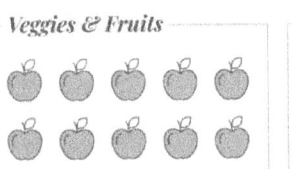

Water

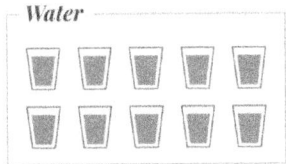

Today's Workout

Stats

Total Calories/Points:

Fat:

Fiber:

Carbs:

Protein:

Exercise:

Sleep:

Notes

Daily Food Diary

Date

Breakfast
Time:

Calories/
Points:

Lunch
Time:

Calories/
Points:

Dinner
Time:

Calories/
Points:

Snack 1
Time:

Calories/
Points:

Snack 2
Time:

Calories/
Points:

Vitamins

Veggies & Fruits

Water

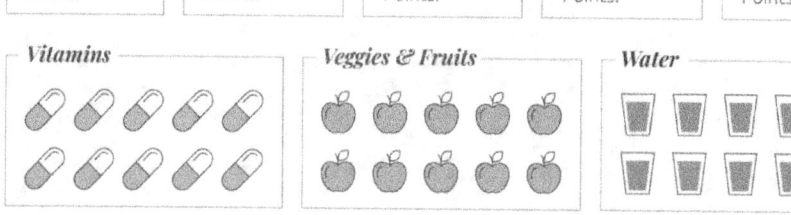

Today's Workout

Stats
Total
Calories/Points:

Fat:

Fiber:

Carbs:

Protein:

Exercise:

Sleep:

Notes

Body PROGRESS

Date							
Weight							
Clothing Size							
Body fat							
Neck							
Chest							
Arms							
Wrists							
Waist							
Hips							
Thighs							
Calfs							
Ankles							

Weight

Date

Daily Food Diary

Breakfast

Time:

Calories/
Points:

Lunch

Time:

Calories/
Points:

Dinner

Time:

Calories/
Points:

Snack 1

Time:

Calories/
Points:

Snack 2

Time:

Calories/
Points:

Vitamins

Veggies & Fruits

Water

Today's Workout

Stats

Total
Calories/Points:

Fat:

Fiber:

Carbs:

Protein:

Exercise:

Sleep:

Notes

Daily Food Diary

Date

Breakfast	Lunch	Dinner	Snack 1	Snack 2
Time:	Time:	Time:	Time:	Time:
Calories/Points:	Calories/Points:	Calories/Points:	Calories/Points:	Calories/Points:

Vitamins

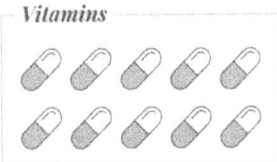

Veggies & Fruits

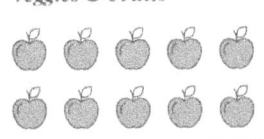

Water

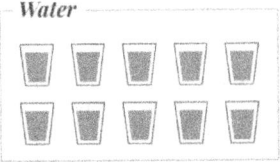

Today's Workout

Stats

Total Calories/Points:

Fat:

Fiber:

Carbs:

Protein:

Exercise:

Sleep:

Notes

Daily Food Diary

Date

Breakfast
Time:

Calories/
Points:

Lunch
Time:

Calories/
Points:

Dinner
Time:

Calories/
Points:

Snack 1
Time:

Calories/
Points:

Snack 2
Time:

Calories/
Points:

Vitamins

Veggies & Fruits

Water

Today's Workout

Stats

Total
Calories/Points:

Fat:

Fiber:

Carbs:

Protein:

Exercise:

Sleep:

Notes

Daily Food Diary

Breakfast	Lunch	Dinner	Snack 1	Snack 2
Time:	Time:	Time:	Time:	Time:
Calories/ Points:	Calories/ Points:	Calories/ Points:	Calories/ Points:	Calories/ Points:

Vitamins

Veggies & Fruits

Water

Today's Workout

Stats

Total Calories/Points:

Fat:

Fiber:

Carbs:

Protein:

Exercise:

Sleep:

Notes

Daily Food Diary

Date

Breakfast
Time:

Calories/
Points:

Lunch
Time:

Calories/
Points:

Dinner
Time:

Calories/
Points:

Snack 1
Time:

Calories/
Points:

Snack 2
Time:

Calories/
Points:

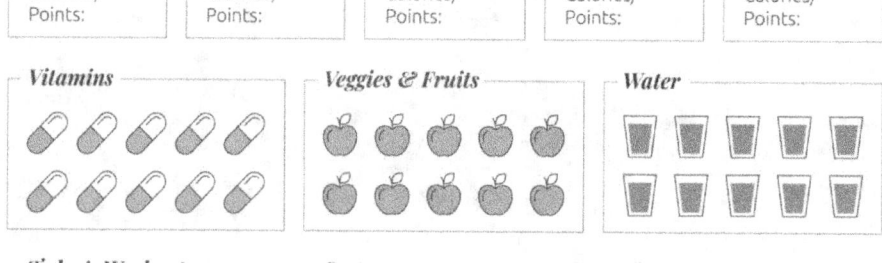

Vitamins

Veggies & Fruits

Water

Today's Workout

Stats

Total
Calories/Points:

Fat:

Fiber:

Carbs:

Protein:

Exercise:

Sleep:

Notes

Daily Food Diary

Date

Breakfast
Time:

Calories/
Points:

Lunch
Time:

Calories/
Points:

Dinner
Time:

Calories/
Points:

Snack 1
Time:

Calories/
Points:

Snack 2
Time:

Calories/
Points:

Vitamins

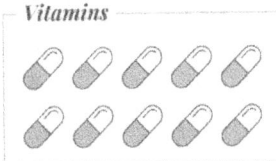

Veggies & Fruits

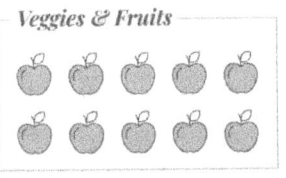

Water

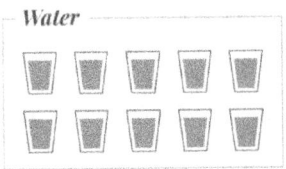

Today's Workout

Stats
Total
Calories/Points:

Fat:

Fiber:

Carbs:

Protein:

Exercise:

Sleep:

Notes

Daily Food Diary

Breakfast
Time:

Calories/
Points:

Lunch
Time:

Calories/
Points:

Dinner
Time:

Calories/
Points:

Snack 1
Time:

Calories/
Points:

Snack 2
Time:

Calories/
Points:

Vitamins

Veggies & Fruits

Water

Today's Workout

Stats
Total
Calories/Points:
Fat:
Fiber:
Carbs:
Protein:
Exercise:
Sleep:

Notes

Body PROGRESS

Date					
Weight					
Clothing Size					
Body fat					
Neck					
Chest					
Arms					
Wrists					
Waist					
Hips					
Thighs					
Calfs					
Ankles					

Weight

Date

Daily Food Diary

Date

Breakfast	*Lunch*	*Dinner*	*Snack 1*	*Snack 2*
Time:	Time:	Time:	Time:	Time:
Calories/ Points:	Calories/ Points:	Calories/ Points:	Calories/ Points:	Calories/ Points:

Vitamins

Veggies & Fruits

Water

Today's Workout

Stats

Total
Calories/Points:

Fat:

Fiber:

Carbs:

Protein:

Exercise:

Sleep:

Notes

Daily Food Diary

Date

Breakfast
Time:

Calories/
Points:

Lunch
Time:

Calories/
Points:

Dinner
Time:

Calories/
Points:

Snack 1
Time:

Calories/
Points:

Snack 2
Time:

Calories/
Points:

Vitamins
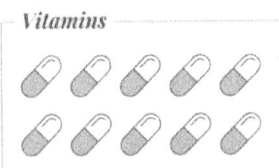

Veggies & Fruits
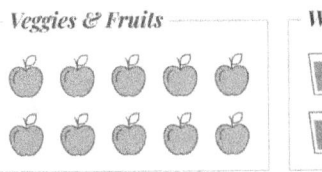

Water
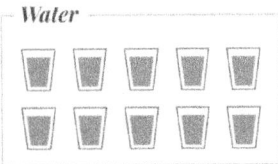

Today's Workout

Stats
Total
Calories/Points:

Fat:

Fiber:

Carbs:

Protein:

Exercise:

Sleep:

Notes

Daily Food Diary

Breakfast
Time:

Calories/
Points:

Lunch
Time:

Calories/
Points:

Dinner
Time:

Calories/
Points:

Snack 1
Time:

Calories/
Points:

Snack 2
Time:

Calories/
Points:

Vitamins

Veggies & Fruits

Water

Today's Workout

Stats
Total
Calories/Points:

Fat:

Fiber:

Carbs:

Protein:

Exercise:

Sleep:

Notes

Daily Food Diary

Date

Breakfast

Time:

Calories/
Points:

Lunch

Time:

Calories/
Points:

Dinner

Time:

Calories/
Points:

Snack 1

Time:

Calories/
Points:

Snack 2

Time:

Calories/
Points:

Vitamins

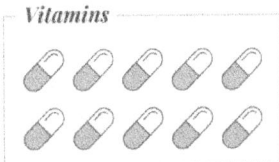

Veggies & Fruits

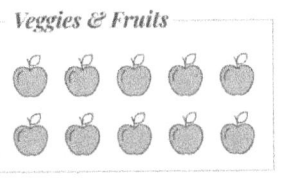

Water

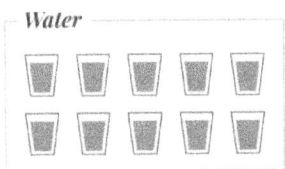

Today's Workout

Stats

Total
Calories/Points:

Fat:

Fiber:

Carbs:

Protein:

Exercise:

Sleep:

Notes

Daily Food Diary

Date

Breakfast
Time:

Calories/
Points:

Lunch
Time:

Calories/
Points:

Dinner
Time:

Calories/
Points:

Snack 1
Time:

Calories/
Points:

Snack 2
Time:

Calories/
Points:

Vitamins

Veggies & Fruits

Water

Today's Workout

Stats

Total
Calories/Points:

Fat:

Fiber:

Carbs:

Protein:

Exercise:

Sleep:

Notes

Daily Food Diary

Date

Breakfast
Time:

Calories/
Points:

Lunch
Time:

Calories/
Points:

Dinner
Time:

Calories/
Points:

Snack 1
Time:

Calories/
Points:

Snack 2
Time:

Calories/
Points:

Vitamins

Veggies & Fruits

Water

Today's Workout

Stats

Total
Calories/Points:

Fat:

Fiber:

Carbs:

Protein:

Exercise:

Sleep:

Notes

Daily Food Diary

Date

Breakfast

Time:

Calories/
Points:

Lunch

Time:

Calories/
Points:

Dinner

Time:

Calories/
Points:

Snack 1

Time:

Calories/
Points:

Snack 2

Time:

Calories/
Points:

Vitamins

Veggies & Fruits

Water

Today's Workout

Stats

Total
Calories/Points:

Fat:

Fiber:

Carbs:

Protein:

Exercise:

Sleep:

Notes

Body PROGRESS

Date						
Weight						
Clothing Size						
Body fat						
Neck						
Chest						
Arms						
Wrists						
Waist						
Hips						
Thighs						
Calfs						
Ankles						

Weight

Date

Daily Food Diary

Breakfast
Time:

Calories/
Points:

Lunch
Time:

Calories/
Points:

Dinner
Time:

Calories/
Points:

Snack 1
Time:

Calories/
Points:

Snack 2
Time:

Calories/
Points:

Vitamins

Veggies & Fruits

Water

Today's Workout

Stats

Total
Calories/Points:

Fat:

Fiber:

Carbs:

Protein:

Exercise:

Sleep:

Notes

Daily Food Diary

Date

Breakfast
Time:

Calories/
Points:

Lunch
Time:

Calories/
Points:

Dinner
Time:

Calories/
Points:

Snack 1
Time:

Calories/
Points:

Snack 2
Time:

Calories/
Points:

Vitamins
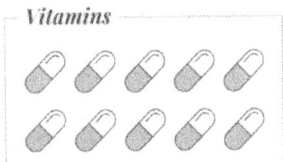

Veggies & Fruits
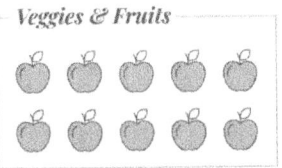

Water
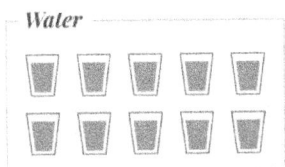

Today's Workout

Stats
Total
Calories/Points:

Fat:

Fiber:

Carbs:

Protein:

Exercise:

Sleep:

Notes

Daily Food Diary

Breakfast
Time:

Calories/
Points:

Lunch
Time:

Calories/
Points:

Dinner
Time:

Calories/
Points:

Snack 1
Time:

Calories/
Points:

Snack 2
Time:

Calories/
Points:

Vitamins

Veggies & Fruits

Water

Today's Workout

Stats
Total
Calories/Points:

Fat:

Fiber:

Carbs:

Protein:

Exercise:

Sleep:

Notes

Daily Food Diary

Date

Breakfast	Lunch	Dinner	Snack 1	Snack 2
Time:	Time:	Time:	Time:	Time:
Calories/ Points:	Calories/ Points:	Calories/ Points:	Calories/ Points:	Calories/ Points:

Vitamins

Veggies & Fruits

Water

Today's Workout

Stats

Total
Calories/Points:

Fat:

Fiber:

Carbs:

Protein:

Exercise:

Sleep:

Notes

Daily Food Diary

Date

Breakfast	Lunch	Dinner	Snack 1	Snack 2
Time:	Time:	Time:	Time:	Time:
Calories/ Points:	Calories/ Points:	Calories/ Points:	Calories/ Points:	Calories/ Points:

Vitamins

Veggies & Fruits

Water

Today's Workout

Stats

Total Calories/Points:

Fat:

Fiber:

Carbs:

Protein:

Exercise:

Sleep:

Notes

Daily Food Diary

Date

Breakfast	Lunch	Dinner	Snack 1	Snack 2
Time:	Time:	Time:	Time:	Time:
Calories/ Points:	Calories/ Points:	Calories/ Points:	Calories/ Points:	Calories/ Points:

Vitamins

Veggies & Fruits

Water

Today's Workout

Stats

Total Calories/Points:

Fat:

Fiber:

Carbs:

Protein:

Exercise:

Sleep:

Notes

Daily Food Diary

Date

Breakfast	Lunch	Dinner	Snack 1	Snack 2
Time:	Time:	Time:	Time:	Time:
Calories/ Points:	Calories/ Points:	Calories/ Points:	Calories/ Points:	Calories/ Points:

Vitamins
Veggies & Fruits
Water

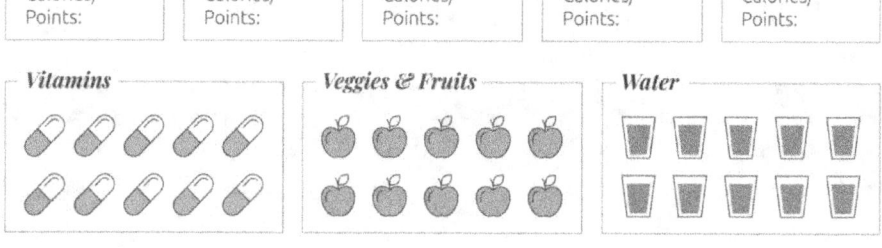

Today's Workout

Stats

Total
Calories/Points:

Fat:

Fiber:

Carbs:

Protein:

Exercise:

Sleep:

Notes

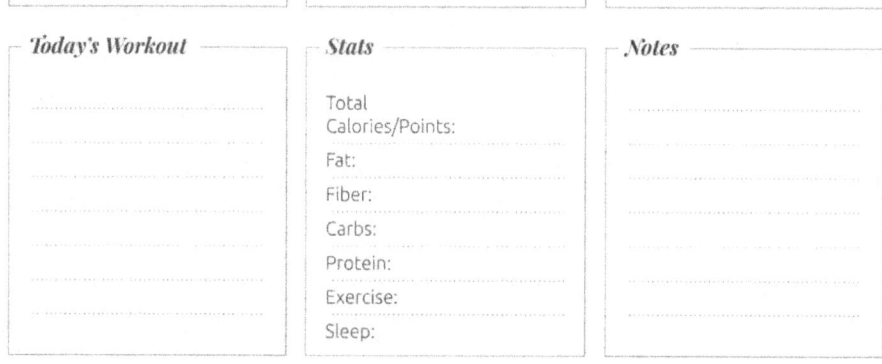

Body PROGRESS

Date							
Weight							
Clothing Size							
Body fat							
Neck							
Chest							
Arms							
Wrists							
Waist							
Hips							
Thighs							
Calfs							
Ankles							

Weight

Date

Daily Food Diary

Date

Breakfast
Time:

Calories/
Points:

Lunch
Time:

Calories/
Points:

Dinner
Time:

Calories/
Points:

Snack 1
Time:

Calories/
Points:

Snack 2
Time:

Calories/
Points:

Vitamins

Veggies & Fruits

Water

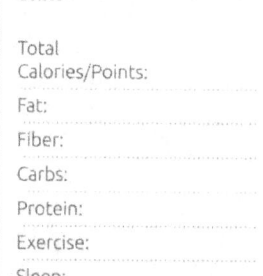

Today's Workout

Stats
Total
Calories/Points:

Fat:

Fiber:

Carbs:

Protein:

Exercise:

Sleep:

Notes

Daily Food Diary

Date

Breakfast	Lunch	Dinner	Snack 1	Snack 2
Time:	Time:	Time:	Time:	Time:
Calories/ Points:	Calories/ Points:	Calories/ Points:	Calories/ Points:	Calories/ Points:

Vitamins

Veggies & Fruits

Water

Today's Workout

Stats

Total
Calories/Points:

Fat:

Fiber:

Carbs:

Protein:

Exercise:

Sleep:

Notes

Daily Food Diary

Date _____

Breakfast	Lunch	Dinner	Snack 1	Snack 2
Time:	Time:	Time:	Time:	Time:
Calories/ Points:	Calories/ Points:	Calories/ Points:	Calories/ Points:	Calories/ Points:

Vitamins

Veggies & Fruits

Water

Today's Workout

Stats

Total
Calories/Points:

Fat:

Fiber:

Carbs:

Protein:

Exercise:

Sleep:

Notes

Daily Food Diary

Date

Breakfast
Time:

Lunch
Time:

Dinner
Time:

Snack 1
Time:

Snack 2
Time:

Calories/
Points:

Calories/
Points:

Calories/
Points:

Calories/
Points:

Calories/
Points:

Vitamins

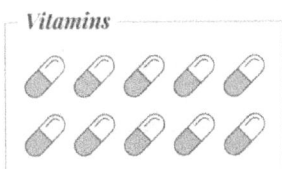

Veggies & Fruits

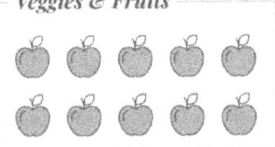

Water

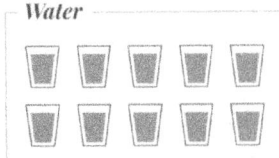

Today's Workout

Stats

Total
Calories/Points:

Fat:

Fiber:

Carbs:

Protein:

Exercise:

Sleep:

Notes

Daily Food Diary

Date

Breakfast

Time:

_____

Calories/
Points:

Lunch

Time:

_____

Calories/
Points:

Dinner

Time:

_____

Calories/
Points:

Snack 1

Time:

_____

Calories/
Points:

Snack 2

Time:

_____

Calories/
Points:

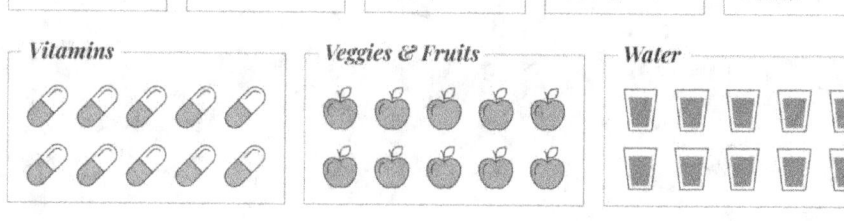

Vitamins

Veggies & Fruits

Water

Today's Workout

Stats

Total
Calories/Points:

Fat:

Fiber:

Carbs:

Protein:

Exercise:

Sleep:

Notes

Daily Food Diary

Date

Breakfast
Time:

Calories/
Points:

Lunch
Time:

Calories/
Points:

Dinner
Time:

Calories/
Points:

Snack 1
Time:

Calories/
Points:

Snack 2
Time:

Calories/
Points:

Vitamins

Veggies & Fruits

Water

Today's Workout

Stats
Total
Calories/Points:

Fat:

Fiber:

Carbs:

Protein:

Exercise:

Sleep:

Notes

Daily Food Diary

Date

Breakfast
Time:

Calories/
Points:

Lunch
Time:

Calories/
Points:

Dinner
Time:

Calories/
Points:

Snack 1
Time:

Calories/
Points:

Snack 2
Time:

Calories/
Points:

Vitamins

Veggies & Fruits

Water

Today's Workout

Stats
Total
Calories/Points:

Fat:

Fiber:

Carbs:

Protein:

Exercise:

Sleep:

Notes

Body PROGRESS

Date						
Weight						
Clothing Size						
Body fat						
Neck						
Chest						
Arms						
Wrists						
Waist						
Hips						
Thighs						
Calfs						
Ankles						

Weight

Date

Daily Food Diary

Breakfast	*Lunch*	*Dinner*	*Snack 1*	*Snack 2*
Time:	Time:	Time:	Time:	Time:
Calories/ Points:	Calories/ Points:	Calories/ Points:	Calories/ Points:	Calories/ Points:

Vitamins

Veggies & Fruits

Water

Today's Workout

Stats

Total
Calories/Points:

Fat:

Fiber:

Carbs:

Protein:

Exercise:

Sleep:

Notes

Daily Food Diary

Date

Breakfast
Time:

Calories/
Points:

Lunch
Time:

Calories/
Points:

Dinner
Time:

Calories/
Points:

Snack 1
Time:

Calories/
Points:

Snack 2
Time:

Calories/
Points:

Vitamins

Veggies & Fruits

Water

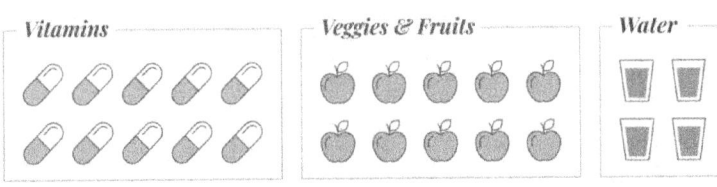

Today's Workout

Stats
Total
Calories/Points:

Fat:

Fiber:

Carbs:

Protein:

Exercise:

Sleep:

Notes

Daily Food Diary

Date

Breakfast
Time:

Calories/
Points:

Lunch
Time:

Calories/
Points:

Dinner
Time:

Calories/
Points:

Snack 1
Time:

Calories/
Points:

Snack 2
Time:

Calories/
Points:

Vitamins

Veggies & Fruits

Water

Today's Workout

Stats

Total
Calories/Points:

Fat:

Fiber:

Carbs:

Protein:

Exercise:

Sleep:

Notes

Daily Food Diary

Date

Breakfast
Time:

Calories/
Points:

Lunch
Time:

Calories/
Points:

Dinner
Time:

Calories/
Points:

Snack 1
Time:

Calories/
Points:

Snack 2
Time:

Calories/
Points:

Vitamins

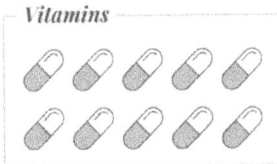

Veggies & Fruits

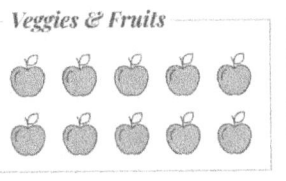

Water

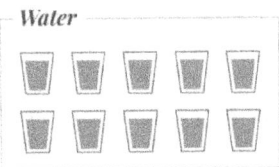

Today's Workout

Stats

Total
Calories/Points:

Fat:

Fiber:

Carbs:

Protein:

Exercise:

Sleep:

Notes

Daily Food Diary

Date

Breakfast	Lunch	Dinner	Snack 1	Snack 2
Time:	Time:	Time:	Time:	Time:
Calories/ Points:	Calories/ Points:	Calories/ Points:	Calories/ Points:	Calories/ Points:

Vitamins

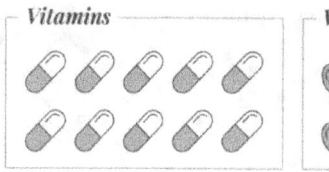

Veggies & Fruits

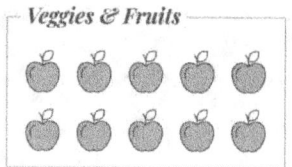

Water

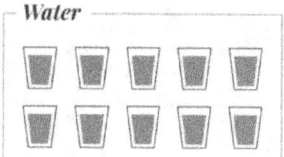

Today's Workout

Stats

Total
Calories/Points:

Fat:

Fiber:

Carbs:

Protein:

Exercise:

Sleep:

Notes

Daily Food Diary

Date _____

Breakfast
Time: _____

Lunch
Time: _____

Dinner
Time: _____

Snack 1
Time: _____

Snack 2
Time: _____

Breakfast Calories/Points: _____

Lunch Calories/Points: _____

Dinner Calories/Points: _____

Snack 1 Calories/Points: _____

Snack 2 Calories/Points: _____

Vitamins

Veggies & Fruits

Water

Today's Workout

Stats

Total Calories/Points: _____

Fat: _____

Fiber: _____

Carbs: _____

Protein: _____

Exercise: _____

Sleep: _____

Notes

Daily Food Diary

Date

Breakfast
Time:

Calories/
Points:

Lunch
Time:

Calories/
Points:

Dinner
Time:

Calories/
Points:

Snack 1
Time:

Calories/
Points:

Snack 2
Time:

Calories/
Points:

Vitamins

Veggies & Fruits

Water

Today's Workout

Stats

Total
Calories/Points:

Fat:

Fiber:

Carbs:

Protein:

Exercise:

Sleep:

Notes

Body PROGRESS

Date						
Weight						
Clothing Size						
Body fat						
Neck						
Chest						
Arms						
Wrists						
Waist						
Hips						
Thighs						
Calfs						
Ankles						

Weight

Date

Daily Food Diary

Breakfast

Time:

Calories/
Points:

Lunch

Time:

Calories/
Points:

Dinner

Time:

Calories/
Points:

Snack 1

Time:

Calories/
Points:

Snack 2

Time:

Calories/
Points:

Vitamins

Veggies & Fruits

Water

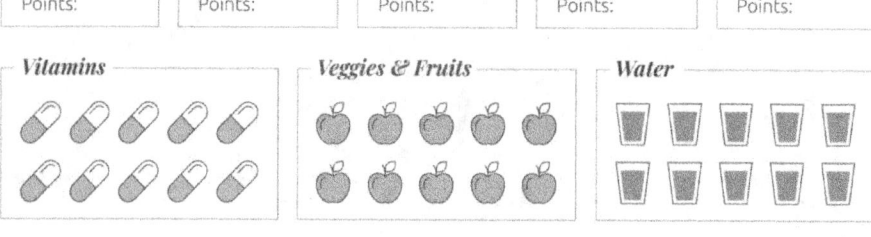

Today's Workout

Stats

Total
Calories/Points:

Fat:

Fiber:

Carbs:

Protein:

Exercise:

Sleep:

Notes

Daily Food Diary

Date

Breakfast	Lunch	Dinner	Snack 1	Snack 2
Time:	Time:	Time:	Time:	Time:

Calories/Points: Calories/Points: Calories/Points: Calories/Points: Calories/Points:

Vitamins

Veggies & Fruits

Water

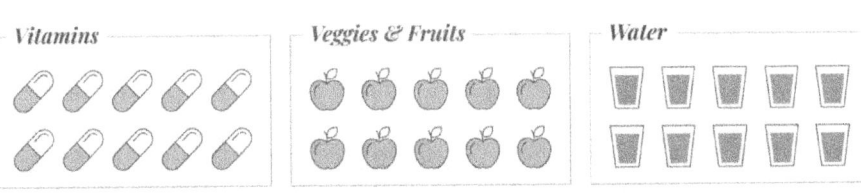

Today's Workout

Stats

Total Calories/Points:

Fat:

Fiber:

Carbs:

Protein:

Exercise:

Sleep:

Notes

Daily Food Diary

Breakfast	Lunch	Dinner	Snack 1	Snack 2
Time:	Time:	Time:	Time:	Time:
Calories/ Points:	Calories/ Points:	Calories/ Points:	Calories/ Points:	Calories/ Points:

Vitamins

Veggies & Fruits

Water

Today's Workout

Stats

Total
Calories/Points:

Fat:

Fiber:

Carbs:

Protein:

Exercise:

Sleep:

Notes

Daily Food Diary

Date

Breakfast	*Lunch*	*Dinner*	*Snack 1*	*Snack 2*
Time:	Time:	Time:	Time:	Time:
Calories/ Points:	Calories/ Points:	Calories/ Points:	Calories/ Points:	Calories/ Points:

Vitamins

Veggies & Fruits

Water

Today's Workout

Stats

Total
Calories/Points:

Fat:

Fiber:

Carbs:

Protein:

Exercise:

Sleep:

Notes

Daily Food Diary

Breakfast
Time:

Calories/
Points:

Lunch
Time:

Calories/
Points:

Dinner
Time:

Calories/
Points:

Snack 1
Time:

Calories/
Points:

Snack 2
Time:

Calories/
Points:

Vitamins

Veggies & Fruits

Water

Today's Workout

Stats

Total
Calories/Points:

Fat:

Fiber:

Carbs:

Protein:

Exercise:

Sleep:

Notes

Daily Food Diary

Date _____

Breakfast	Lunch	Dinner	Snack 1	Snack 2
Time:	Time:	Time:	Time:	Time:
Calories/ Points:	Calories/ Points:	Calories/ Points:	Calories/ Points:	Calories/ Points:

Vitamins

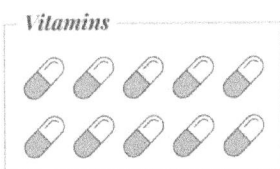

Veggies & Fruits

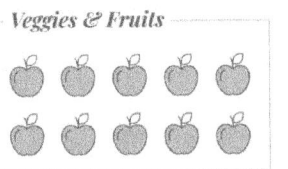

Water

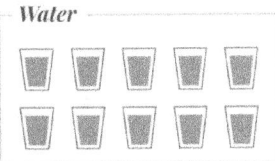

Today's Workout

_____

Stats

Total Calories/Points:

Fat:

Fiber:

Carbs:

Protein:

Exercise:

Sleep:

Notes

Daily Food Diary

Breakfast	Lunch	Dinner	Snack 1	Snack 2
Time:	Time:	Time:	Time:	Time:
Calories/ Points:	Calories/ Points:	Calories/ Points:	Calories/ Points:	Calories/ Points:

Vitamins

Veggies & Fruits

Water

Today's Workout

Stats

Total
Calories/Points:

Fat:

Fiber:

Carbs:

Protein:

Exercise:

Sleep:

Notes

Body PROGRESS

Date							
Weight							
Clothing Size							
Body fat							
Neck							
Chest							
Arms							
Wrists							
Waist							
Hips							
Thighs							
Calfs							
Ankles							

Weight

Date

Daily Food Diary

Date

Breakfast
Time:

Calories/
Points:

Lunch
Time:

Calories/
Points:

Dinner
Time:

Calories/
Points:

Snack 1
Time:

Calories/
Points:

Snack 2
Time:

Calories/
Points:

Vitamins

Veggies & Fruits

Water

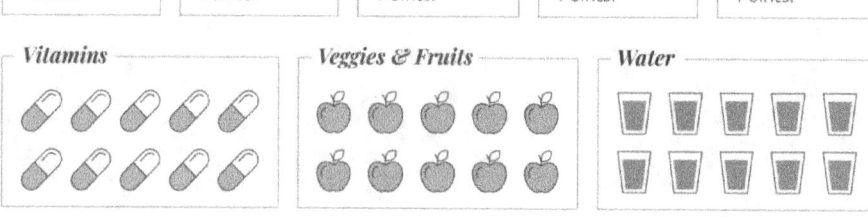

Today's Workout

Stats

Total
Calories/Points:

Fat:

Fiber:

Carbs:

Protein:

Exercise:

Sleep:

Notes

Daily Food Diary

Date

Breakfast
Time:

Calories/
Points:

Lunch
Time:

Calories/
Points:

Dinner
Time:

Calories/
Points:

Snack 1
Time:

Calories/
Points:

Snack 2
Time:

Calories/
Points:

Vitamins

Veggies & Fruits

Water

Today's Workout

Stats

Total
Calories/Points:

Fat:

Fiber:

Carbs:

Protein:

Exercise:

Sleep:

Notes

Daily Food Diary

Breakfast	*Lunch*	*Dinner*	*Snack 1*	*Snack 2*
Time:	Time:	Time:	Time:	Time:
Calories/ Points:	Calories/ Points:	Calories/ Points:	Calories/ Points:	Calories/ Points:

Vitamins

Veggies & Fruits

Water

Today's Workout

Stats

Total
Calories/Points:

Fat:

Fiber:

Carbs:

Protein:

Exercise:

Sleep:

Notes

Daily Food Diary

Date _____

Breakfast
Time: _____

_____
_____
_____
_____
_____
_____
_____
_____
_____
_____
_____
_____
_____
_____
_____
_____

Calories/
Points:

Lunch
Time: _____

_____
_____
_____
_____
_____
_____
_____
_____
_____
_____
_____
_____
_____
_____
_____
_____

Calories/
Points:

Dinner
Time: _____

_____
_____
_____
_____
_____
_____
_____
_____
_____
_____
_____
_____
_____
_____
_____
_____

Calories/
Points:

Snack 1
Time: _____

_____
_____
_____
_____
_____
_____
_____
_____
_____
_____
_____
_____
_____

Calories/
Points:

Snack 2
Time: _____

_____
_____
_____
_____
_____
_____
_____
_____
_____
_____
_____
_____
_____

Calories/
Points:

Vitamins
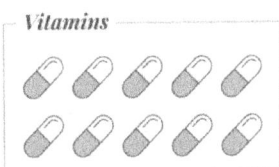

Veggies & Fruits
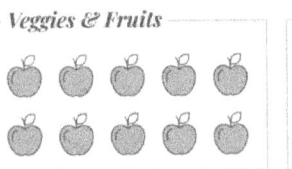

Water
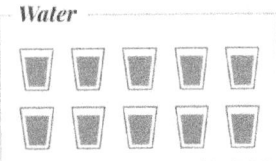

Today's Workout

_____
_____
_____
_____
_____
_____
_____

Stats

Total
Calories/Points:

Fat:

Fiber:

Carbs:

Protein:

Exercise:

Sleep:

Notes

_____
_____
_____
_____
_____
_____
_____

Daily Food Diary

Breakfast

Time:

Calories/
Points:

Lunch

Time:

Calories/
Points:

Dinner

Time:

Calories/
Points:

Snack 1

Time:

Calories/
Points:

Snack 2

Time:

Calories/
Points:

Vitamins

Veggies & Fruits

Water

Today's Workout

Stats

Total
Calories/Points:

Fat:

Fiber:

Carbs:

Protein:

Exercise:

Sleep:

Notes

Daily Food Diary

Breakfast
Time:

Calories/
Points:

Lunch
Time:

Calories/
Points:

Dinner
Time:

Calories/
Points:

Snack 1
Time:

Calories/
Points:

Snack 2
Time:

Calories/
Points:

Vitamins

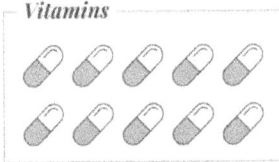

Veggies & Fruits

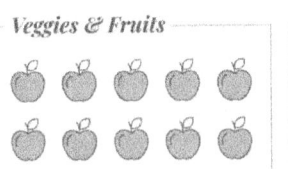

Water

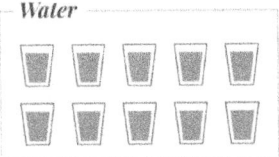

Today's Workout

Stats

Total
Calories/Points:

Fat:

Fiber:

Carbs:

Protein:

Exercise:

Sleep:

Notes

Daily Food Diary

Date

Breakfast
Time:

Calories/
Points:

Lunch
Time:

Calories/
Points:

Dinner
Time:

Calories/
Points:

Snack 1
Time:

Calories/
Points:

Snack 2
Time:

Calories/
Points:

Vitamins

Veggies & Fruits

Water

Today's Workout

Stats

Total
Calories/Points:

Fat:

Fiber:

Carbs:

Protein:

Exercise:

Sleep:

Notes

Body PROGRESS

Date							
Weight							
Clothing Size							
Body fat							
Neck							
Chest							
Arms							
Wrists							
Waist							
Hips							
Thighs							
Calfs							
Ankles							

Weight

Date

Daily Food Diary

Date

Breakfast
Time:

Calories/
Points:

Lunch
Time:

Calories/
Points:

Dinner
Time:

Calories/
Points:

Snack 1
Time:

Calories/
Points:

Snack 2
Time:

Calories/
Points:

Vitamins

Veggies & Fruits

Water

Today's Workout

Stats

Total
Calories/Points:

Fat:

Fiber:

Carbs:

Protein:

Exercise:

Sleep:

Notes

Daily Food Diary

Date

Breakfast
Time:

Calories/
Points:

Lunch
Time:

Calories/
Points:

Dinner
Time:

Calories/
Points:

Snack 1
Time:

Calories/
Points:

Snack 2
Time:

Calories/
Points:

Vitamins
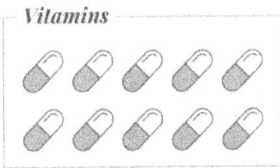

Veggies & Fruits
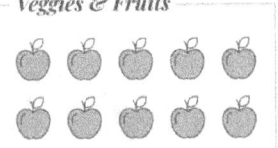

Water
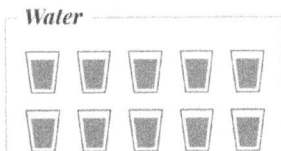

Today's Workout

Stats
Total
Calories/Points:

Fat:

Fiber:

Carbs:

Protein:

Exercise:

Sleep:

Notes

Daily Food Diary

Breakfast
Time:

Calories/
Points:

Lunch
Time:

Calories/
Points:

Dinner
Time:

Calories/
Points:

Snack 1
Time:

Calories/
Points:

Snack 2
Time:

Calories/
Points:

Vitamins

Veggies & Fruits

Water

Today's Workout

Stats

Total
Calories/Points:

Fat:

Fiber:

Carbs:

Protein:

Exercise:

Sleep:

Notes

Daily Food Diary

Breakfast	*Lunch*	*Dinner*	*Snack 1*	*Snack 2*
Time:	Time:	Time:	Time:	Time:
Calories/ Points:	Calories/ Points:	Calories/ Points:	Calories/ Points:	Calories/ Points:

Vitamins

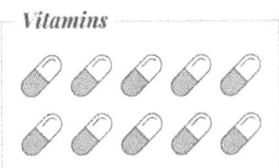

Veggies & Fruits

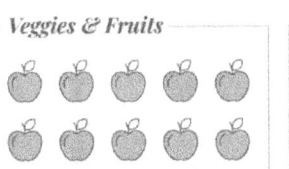

Water

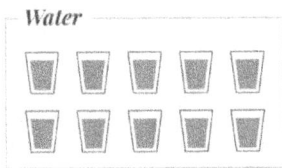

Today's Workout

Stats

Total Calories/Points:

Fat:

Fiber:

Carbs:

Protein:

Exercise:

Sleep:

Notes

Daily Food Diary

Date

Breakfast
Time:

Calories/
Points:

Lunch
Time:

Calories/
Points:

Dinner
Time:

Calories/
Points:

Snack 1
Time:

Calories/
Points:

Snack 2
Time:

Calories/
Points:

Vitamins

Veggies & Fruits

Water

Today's Workout

Stats
Total
Calories/Points:

Fat:

Fiber:

Carbs:

Protein:

Exercise:

Sleep:

Notes

Daily Food Diary

Date

Breakfast
Time:

Calories/
Points:

Lunch
Time:

Calories/
Points:

Dinner
Time:

Calories/
Points:

Snack 1
Time:

Calories/
Points:

Snack 2
Time:

Calories/
Points:

Vitamins

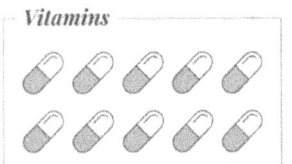

Veggies & Fruits

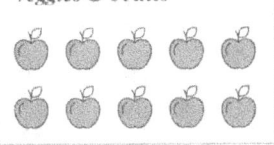

Water

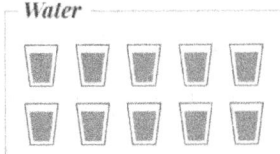

Today's Workout

Stats

Total
Calories/Points:

Fat:

Fiber:

Carbs:

Protein:

Exercise:

Sleep:

Notes

Daily Food Diary

Breakfast
Time:

Calories/
Points:

Lunch
Time:

Calories/
Points:

Dinner
Time:

Calories/
Points:

Snack 1
Time:

Calories/
Points:

Snack 2
Time:

Calories/
Points:

Vitamins

Veggies & Fruits

Water

Today's Workout

Stats

Total
Calories/Points:

Fat:

Fiber:

Carbs:

Protein:

Exercise:

Sleep:

Notes

Body PROGRESS

Date							
Weight							
Clothing Size							
Body fat							
Neck							
Chest							
Arms							
Wrists							
Waist							
Hips							
Thighs							
Calfs							
Ankles							

Weight

Date

Daily Food Diary

Breakfast
Time:

Calories/
Points:

Lunch
Time:

Calories/
Points:

Dinner
Time:

Calories/
Points:

Snack 1
Time:

Calories/
Points:

Snack 2
Time:

Calories/
Points:

Vitamins

Veggies & Fruits

Water

Today's Workout

Stats

Total
Calories/Points:

Fat:

Fiber:

Carbs:

Protein:

Exercise:

Sleep:

Notes

Daily Food Diary

Date

Breakfast
Time:

Calories/
Points:

Lunch
Time:

Calories/
Points:

Dinner
Time:

Calories/
Points:

Snack 1
Time:

Calories/
Points:

Snack 2
Time:

Calories/
Points:

Vitamins

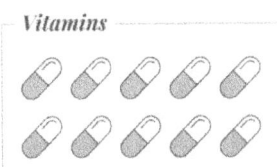

Veggies & Fruits

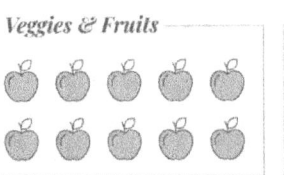

Water

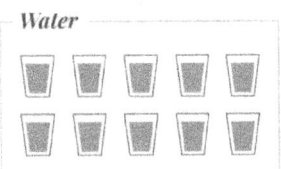

Today's Workout

Stats

Total
Calories/Points:

Fat:

Fiber:

Carbs:

Protein:

Exercise:

Sleep:

Notes

Daily Food Diary

Date

Breakfast

Time:

_____

Calories/
Points:

Lunch

Time:

_____

Calories/
Points:

Dinner

Time:

_____

Calories/
Points:

Snack 1

Time:

_____

Calories/
Points:

Snack 2

Time:

_____

Calories/
Points:

Vitamins

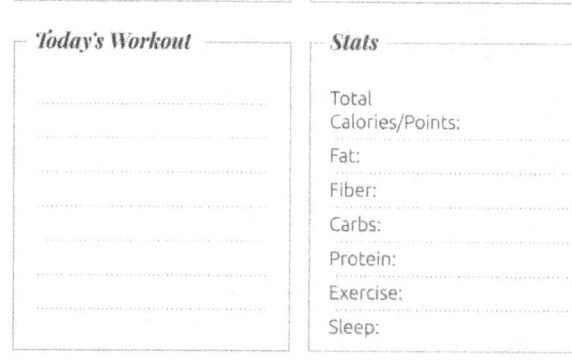

Veggies & Fruits

Water

Today's Workout

_____

Stats

Total
Calories/Points:

Fat:

Fiber:

Carbs:

Protein:

Exercise:

Sleep:

Notes

_____

Daily Food Diary

Breakfast	Lunch	Dinner	Snack 1	Snack 2
Time:	Time:	Time:	Time:	Time:
Calories/ Points:	Calories/ Points:	Calories/ Points:	Calories/ Points:	Calories/ Points:

Vitamins

Veggies & Fruits

Water

Today's Workout

Stats

Total
Calories/Points:

Fat:

Fiber:

Carbs:

Protein:

Exercise:

Sleep:

Notes

Daily Food Diary

Date

Breakfast
Time:

Calories/
Points:

Lunch
Time:

Calories/
Points:

Dinner
Time:

Calories/
Points:

Snack 1
Time:

Calories/
Points:

Snack 2
Time:

Calories/
Points:

Vitamins

Veggies & Fruits

Water

Today's Workout

Stats
Total
Calories/Points:

Fat:

Fiber:

Carbs:

Protein:

Exercise:

Sleep:

Notes

Daily Food Diary

Date

Breakfast
Time:

Calories/
Points:

Lunch
Time:

Calories/
Points:

Dinner
Time:

Calories/
Points:

Snack 1
Time:

Calories/
Points:

Snack 2
Time:

Calories/
Points:

Vitamins

Veggies & Fruits

Water

Today's Workout

Stats

Total
Calories/Points:

Fat:

Fiber:

Carbs:

Protein:

Exercise:

Sleep:

Notes

Daily Food Diary

Date

Breakfast	*Lunch*	*Dinner*	*Snack 1*	*Snack 2*
Time:	Time:	Time:	Time:	Time:
Calories/Points:	Calories/Points:	Calories/Points:	Calories/Points:	Calories/Points:

Vitamins

Veggies & Fruits

Water

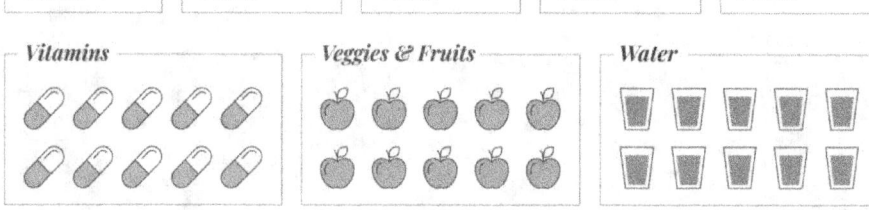

Today's Workout

Stats

Total
Calories/Points:

Fat:

Fiber:

Carbs:

Protein:

Exercise:

Sleep:

Notes

Body PROGRESS

Date							
Weight							
Clothing Size							
Body fat							
Neck							
Chest							
Arms							
Wrists							
Waist							
Hips							
Thighs							
Calfs							
Ankles							

Weight

Date

Daily Food Diary

Breakfast

Time:

_____

Calories/
Points:

Lunch

Time:

_____

Calories/
Points:

Dinner

Time:

_____

Calories/
Points:

Snack 1

Time:

_____

Calories/
Points:

Snack 2

Time:

_____

Calories/
Points:

Vitamins

Veggies & Fruits

Water

Today's Workout

Stats

Total
Calories/Points:

Fat:

Fiber:

Carbs:

Protein:

Exercise:

Sleep:

Notes

Daily Food Diary

Date

Breakfast
Time:

Calories/
Points:

Lunch
Time:

Calories/
Points:

Dinner
Time:

Calories/
Points:

Snack 1
Time:

Calories/
Points:

Snack 2
Time:

Calories/
Points:

Vitamins

Veggies & Fruits

Water

Today's Workout

Stats

Total
Calories/Points:

Fat:

Fiber:

Carbs:

Protein:

Exercise:

Sleep:

Notes

Daily Food Diary

Date

Breakfast	*Lunch*	*Dinner*	*Snack 1*	*Snack 2*
Time:	Time:	Time:	Time:	Time:
Calories/ Points:	Calories/ Points:	Calories/ Points:	Calories/ Points:	Calories/ Points:

Vitamins

Veggies & Fruits

Water

Today's Workout

Stats

Total
Calories/Points:

Fat:

Fiber:

Carbs:

Protein:

Exercise:

Sleep:

Notes

Daily Food Diary

Date

Breakfast
Time:

Calories/
Points:

Lunch
Time:

Calories/
Points:

Dinner
Time:

Calories/
Points:

Snack 1
Time:

Calories/
Points:

Snack 2
Time:

Calories/
Points:

Vitamins

Veggies & Fruits

Water

Today's Workout

Stats

Total
Calories/Points:

Fat:

Fiber:

Carbs:

Protein:

Exercise:

Sleep:

Notes

Daily Food Diary

Date

Breakfast	Lunch	Dinner	Snack 1	Snack 2
Time:	Time:	Time:	Time:	Time:
Calories/ Points:	Calories/ Points:	Calories/ Points:	Calories/ Points:	Calories/ Points:

Vitamins

Veggies & Fruits

Water

Today's Workout

Stats

Total
Calories/Points:

Fat:

Fiber:

Carbs:

Protein:

Exercise:

Sleep:

Notes

Daily Food Diary

Date

Breakfast
Time:

Calories/
Points:

Lunch
Time:

Calories/
Points:

Dinner
Time:

Calories/
Points:

Snack 1
Time:

Calories/
Points:

Snack 2
Time:

Calories/
Points:

Vitamins

Veggies & Fruits

Water

Today's Workout

Stats

Total
Calories/Points:

Fat:

Fiber:

Carbs:

Protein:

Exercise:

Sleep:

Notes

Daily Food Diary

Breakfast
Time:

Calories/
Points:

Lunch
Time:

Calories/
Points:

Dinner
Time:

Calories/
Points:

Snack 1
Time:

Calories/
Points:

Snack 2
Time:

Calories/
Points:

Vitamins

Veggies & Fruits

Water

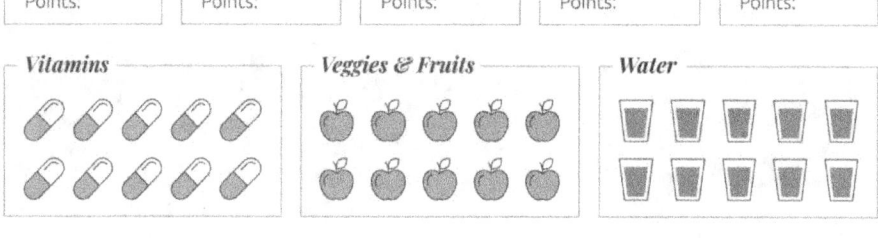

Today's Workout

Stats
Total
Calories/Points:

Fat:

Fiber:

Carbs:

Protein:

Exercise:

Sleep:

Notes

Body PROGRESS

Date							
Weight							
Clothing Size							
Body fat							
Neck							
Chest							
Arms							
Wrists							
Waist							
Hips							
Thighs							
Calfs							
Ankles							

Weight

Date

Daily Food Diary

Date

Breakfast

Time:

....
....
....
....
....
....
....
....
....
....
....
....
....
....
....
....

Calories/
Points:

Lunch

Time:

....
....
....
....
....
....
....
....
....
....
....
....
....
....
....
....

Calories/
Points:

Dinner

Time:

....
....
....
....
....
....
....
....
....
....
....
....
....
....
....
....

Calories/
Points:

Snack 1

Time:

....
....
....
....
....
....
....
....
....
....
....
....
....
....
....
....

Calories/
Points:

Snack 2

Time:

....
....
....
....
....
....
....
....
....
....
....
....
....
....
....
....

Calories/
Points:

Vitamins

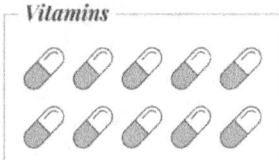

Veggies & Fruits

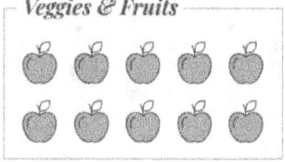

Water

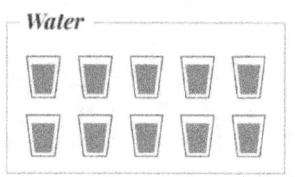

Today's Workout

....
....
....
....
....
....

Stats

Total
Calories/Points:

Fat:

Fiber:

Carbs:

Protein:

Exercise:

Sleep:

Notes

....
....
....
....
....

Daily Food Diary

Date _____

Breakfast	*Lunch*	*Dinner*	*Snack 1*	*Snack 2*
Time:	Time:	Time:	Time:	Time:
Calories/ Points:	Calories/ Points:	Calories/ Points:	Calories/ Points:	Calories/ Points:

Vitamins

Veggies & Fruits

Water

Today's Workout

Stats

Total Calories/Points:

Fat:

Fiber:

Carbs:

Protein:

Exercise:

Sleep:

Notes

Daily Food Diary

Date

Breakfast
Time:

Calories/
Points:

Lunch
Time:

Calories/
Points:

Dinner
Time:

Calories/
Points:

Snack 1
Time:

Calories/
Points:

Snack 2
Time:

Calories/
Points:

Vitamins

Veggies & Fruits

Water

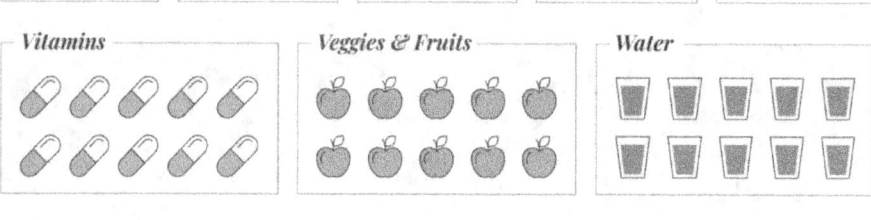

Today's Workout

Stats

Total
Calories/Points:

Fat:

Fiber:

Carbs:

Protein:

Exercise:

Sleep:

Notes

Daily Food Diary

Breakfast
Time:

Calories/
Points:

Lunch
Time:

Calories/
Points:

Dinner
Time:

Calories/
Points:

Snack 1
Time:

Calories/
Points:

Snack 2
Time:

Calories/
Points:

Vitamins

Veggies & Fruits

Water

Today's Workout

Stats
Total
Calories/Points:

Fat:

Fiber:

Carbs:

Protein:

Exercise:

Sleep:

Notes

Daily Food Diary

Breakfast
Time:

Calories/
Points:

Lunch
Time:

Calories/
Points:

Dinner
Time:

Calories/
Points:

Snack 1
Time:

Calories/
Points:

Snack 2
Time:

Calories/
Points:

Vitamins

Veggies & Fruits

Water

Today's Workout

Stats

Total
Calories/Points:

Fat:

Fiber:

Carbs:

Protein:

Exercise:

Sleep:

Notes

Daily Food Diary

Breakfast
Time:

Calories/
Points:

Lunch
Time:

Calories/
Points:

Dinner
Time:

Calories/
Points:

Snack 1
Time:

Calories/
Points:

Snack 2
Time:

Calories/
Points:

Vitamins

Veggies & Fruits

Water

Today's Workout

Stats

Total
Calories/Points:

Fat:

Fiber:

Carbs:

Protein:

Exercise:

Sleep:

Notes

Daily Food Diary

Date _____

Breakfast
Time:
_____

Calories/
Points:

Lunch
Time:
_____

Calories/
Points:

Dinner
Time:
_____

Calories/
Points:

Snack 1
Time:
_____

Calories/
Points:

Snack 2
Time:
_____

Calories/
Points:

Vitamins

Veggies & Fruits

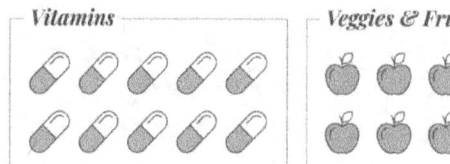

Water

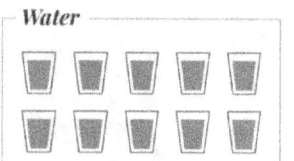

Today's Workout

Stats

Total
Calories/Points:

Fat:

Fiber:

Carbs:

Protein:

Exercise:

Sleep:

Notes

Body PROGRESS

Date							
Weight							
Clothing Size							
Body fat							
Neck							
Chest							
Arms							
Wrists							
Waist							
Hips							
Thighs							
Calfs							
Ankles							

Weight

Date

Daily Food Diary

Date

Breakfast
Time:

Calories/
Points:

Lunch
Time:

Calories/
Points:

Dinner
Time:

Calories/
Points:

Snack 1
Time:

Calories/
Points:

Snack 2
Time:

Calories/
Points:

Vitamins

Veggies & Fruits

Water

Today's Workout

Stats

Total
Calories/Points:

Fat:

Fiber:

Carbs:

Protein:

Exercise:

Sleep:

Notes

Daily Food Diary

Breakfast
Time:

Calories/
Points:

Lunch
Time:

Calories/
Points:

Dinner
Time:

Calories/
Points:

Snack 1
Time:

Calories/
Points:

Snack 2
Time:

Calories/
Points:

Vitamins

Veggies & Fruits

Water

Today's Workout

Stats

Total
Calories/Points:

Fat:

Fiber:

Carbs:

Protein:

Exercise:

Sleep:

Notes

Daily Food Diary

Breakfast

Time:

Calories/
Points:

Lunch

Time:

Calories/
Points:

Dinner

Time:

Calories/
Points:

Snack 1

Time:

Calories/
Points:

Snack 2

Time:

Calories/
Points:

Vitamins

Veggies & Fruits

Water

Today's Workout

Stats

Total
Calories/Points:

Fat:

Fiber:

Carbs:

Protein:

Exercise:

Sleep:

Notes

Daily Food Diary

Date _____

Breakfast
Time: _____

_____
_____
_____
_____
_____
_____
_____
_____
_____
_____
_____
_____
_____
_____

Calories/
Points:

Lunch
Time: _____

_____
_____
_____
_____
_____
_____
_____
_____
_____
_____
_____
_____
_____
_____

Calories/
Points:

Dinner
Time: _____

_____
_____
_____
_____
_____
_____
_____
_____
_____
_____
_____
_____
_____
_____

Calories/
Points:

Snack 1
Time: _____

_____
_____
_____
_____
_____
_____
_____
_____
_____
_____
_____
_____
_____
_____

Calories/
Points:

Snack 2
Time: _____

_____
_____
_____
_____
_____
_____
_____
_____
_____
_____
_____
_____
_____
_____

Calories/
Points:

Vitamins

Veggies & Fruits

Water

Today's Workout

_____
_____
_____
_____
_____
_____
_____

Stats

Total
Calories/Points:

Fat:

Fiber:

Carbs:

Protein:

Exercise:

Sleep:

Notes

_____
_____
_____
_____
_____
_____

Daily Food Diary

Date _____

Breakfast	Lunch	Dinner	Snack 1	Snack 2
Time:	Time:	Time:	Time:	Time:
Calories/ Points:	Calories/ Points:	Calories/ Points:	Calories/ Points:	Calories/ Points:

Vitamins

Veggies & Fruits

Water

Today's Workout

Stats

Total
Calories/Points:

Fat:

Fiber:

Carbs:

Protein:

Exercise:

Sleep:

Notes

Daily Food Diary

Breakfast	*Lunch*	*Dinner*	*Snack 1*	*Snack 2*
Time:	Time:	Time:	Time:	Time:
Calories/ Points:	Calories/ Points:	Calories/ Points:	Calories/ Points:	Calories/ Points:

Vitamins

Veggies & Fruits

Water

Today's Workout

Stats

Total Calories/Points:

Fat:

Fiber:

Carbs:

Protein:

Exercise:

Sleep:

Notes

Daily Food Diary

Date _____

Breakfast	Lunch	Dinner	Snack 1	Snack 2
Time:	Time:	Time:	Time:	Time:

Calories/Points: _____ | Calories/Points: _____ | Calories/Points: _____ | Calories/Points: _____ | Calories/Points: _____

Vitamins

Veggies & Fruits

Water

Today's Workout

Stats

Total Calories/Points:

Fat:

Fiber:

Carbs:

Protein:

Exercise:

Sleep:

Notes

Body PROGRESS

Date						
Weight						
Clothing Size						
Body fat						
Neck						
Chest						
Arms						
Wrists						
Waist						
Hips						
Thighs						
Calfs						
Ankles						

Weight

Date